Katherine Ponte

Foreword by
Joseph F. Goldberg, M.D.

THE Bipolar CHECKLIST

"

What to do
when it matters most

A REAL-TIME ACTION GUIDE FOR CAREGIVERS

To Izzy,
for showing me that love is stronger than bipolar.

AUTHOR'S NOTE

This publication is provided for general informational and educational purposes only. It is not a substitute for medical, mental health, legal, financial, or other professional advice, diagnosis, or treatment. Always consult an appropriately qualified healthcare provider or other competent professional regarding your individual circumstances.

www.katherineponte.com

FOREWORD

Caregivers who have a loved one with bipolar disorder face enormous challenges in navigating the complexities of this disorder. Bipolar disorder is, for most people, a chronic and lifelong condition (like hypertension or heart disease) that requires management, education, and support to achieve not just symptom control, but a sense of normalcy over everyday life. Caregivers play a crucial role in this process. On the one hand, they are the first-line "responders" and supports for their loved ones who may need help in ways they might not fully realize; caregivers function as advocates, guardians, lookouts, and partners for helping their loved one maintain the best life they can. At the same time, caregivers run the risk of losing sight of their own needs, feeling alienation, facing a sense of loss or confusion, or not knowing what to do when they need answers to immediate questions.

Here, now, at long last, caregivers have a place to turn for concise practical guidance about what to expect, and what to do, when they face the challenges and uncertainties of caring for a loved one with bipolar disorder. Katherine Ponte has developed an innovative, to-the-point, highly practical roadmap, informed by lived experience as well as her own scholarship as a psychiatric academician and mental health recovery expert. She tackles the most pressing, and at times vexing, situations that might otherwise leave even the most compassionate and dedicated family members or significant others baffled about what to do in the face of relapse, residual symptoms, problems functioning in life, procuring appropriate healthcare, or managing interpersonal conflicts. Herein, she lays out a roadmap that can help caregivers recognize and understand symptoms, triggers, and resources, and find ways to develop action plans before they're needed. How can they help tackle poor treatment adherence? How should they recognize and respond to a loved one's lack of insight, or denial of illness, as a cognitive sign of the illness itself? How can they defuse arguments in the face of undertreated symptoms, and foster the best possible kinds of communication styles? What is the role of peer support? What is the right level of care for a given level of symptoms? How can they best help their loved one engage their treatment provider, or treatment team, to avert crises before they happen—and how can they know exactly what to do when even the best-laid plans fall short.

I know of few other resources available to patients and their families or significant others that provide such immediate guidance. Katherine successfully aims to capture, in a no-nonsense, simple-language, direct and easy-to-follow format, a how-to guide that bridges the gap between knowledge and action. Her guidance can facilitate real-time decision-making and instill a greater sense of confidence in how to best manage this complex, often hard-to-treat mental health condition in order to help their loved ones reach true recovery – that is, the ability to regain a sense of their lives as whole, thriving individuals – with maximum success.

Joseph F. Goldberg, M.D.
Clinical Professor of Psychiatry
Icahn School of Medicine at Mount Sinai, New York, NY
Immediate-Past President, American Society of Clinical Psychopharmacology
Deputy Editor-in-Chief, The Journal of Clinical Psychiatry

ENDORSEMENTS

This is an excellent resource for loved ones that want to know how to approach their loved one with a complex and at times confusing condition. The Checklist is based on Katherine's own valuable personal experience, and this shows. I highly recommend this resource to help approach this important challenge. Recovery is possible and following this will help promote that.

Ken Duckworth, MD
Retired Chief Medical Officer of NAMI National
Assistant Professor of Psychiatry, Harvard Medical School

The Bipolar Checklist is extraordinary because it fills a desperate need for families - practical, compassionate, real-time guidance to navigate crises, reduce conflict, and support recovery. Katherine combines lived experience, deep knowledge of mental health systems, and genuine empathy to deliver guidance that is actionable and grounded in the reality that recovery is possible.

I believe this book will become an invaluable resource for caregivers, families, advocates, and anyone supporting a loved one with bipolar disorder. As someone raised by a mother with severe bipolar disorder, I wish my family such a resource.

Nathan Romano, MBA
President Emeritus of NAMI-NYC
Board Member of NAMI National

As a NAMI Family-to-Family instructor and caregiver, I've seen how challenging it can be to know what to do in the moment. This book fills that gap. It's clear, practical, and grounded in real experience—offering step-by-step guidance when caregivers need it most. I'll be recommending this to the families I work with.

John De Natale, LMSW
Family-to-Family Instructor of NAMI-NYC
Former Board Member of NAMI-NYC

THE BIPOLAR CHECKLIST

A Real-Time Action Guide for Caregivers

When someone you love is living with bipolar disorder, things can change quickly and without warning.

What felt manageable yesterday can suddenly feel overwhelming, confusing, or even frightening. You may not know what to do next. Acting quickly matters. Early intervention can help prevent symptoms from worsening, make a condition easier to treat, and reduce suffering.

In those moments, the hardest question is often the simplest: What do I do right now?

The Bipolar Checklist is a real-time, action-oriented tool for caregivers, designed for moments when clarity matters most. It is grounded in lived experience and clinical insight.

Use alongside, not instead of, clinical care. For deeper understanding, resources such as *Loving Someone with a Serious Mental Illness* can provide a more comprehensive foundation.

Recovery is possible. And you don't have to navigate this alone.

You don't need to understand everything.
You need to know what to do next, right now.

Start where you are.
Take the next step.

Start here.

HOW TO USE THIS CHECKLIST

☐ Go to Part I: Quick Start for immediate actions based on what's happening to you now
☐ Use during uncertainty
☐ Act now if safety is a concern
☐ Follow the "Go To" instructions
☐ Go to different section of the book when guided

This checklist offers guidance, not rules.

Every situation is different. If something doesn't fit, you are not failing. Use your judgment. Some things may not be possible and that's okay.

Table of Contents

PART I: QUICK START

PART II: WHAT TO KNOW

1. Understanding Bipolar Disorder 9
2. Resources & Education 13
3. Types of Hospitalization 14
4. Insurance 15
5. Treatment Team 16
6. Medication & Non-Therapy Treatments 19
7. Therapy Options and Other 21
8. Community-Based Services 22
9. Psychoeducation 23
10. Health Risks & Monitoring 23
11. Peer Support & Community 24
12. Emotional Support Animals (ESAs) 25
13. Privacy & Legal (HIPAA) 26
14. Government Benefits (think long term) 27

PART III: WHAT TO DO

1. Understanding their Experience 31
2. If Your Loved One Shows Symptoms of Mania or Hypomania 33
3. If Your Loved One Shows Symptoms of Depression 35
4. When Cognitive Impairments are Emerging 38
5. When Psychosis is Emerging 38
6. Crisis & Immediate Safety 39
7. When They Are Not a Danger but Clearly Unwell 42
8. Suicide Risk & Prevention 45

9. Screening & Starting Treatment 46
10. When They Refuse Help 53
11. Reducing Conflict & De-escalation 55
12. What To Do After a Crisis 56
13. Boundaries 57
14. Crisis Planning & Higher Levels of Care 59
15. How to Communicate 61
16. Monitoring & Prevention 63
17. Ready to Pursue Recovery? 67
18. Healthy Lifestyle 69
19. Routine & Environment 73
20. Community & Functional Life 75
21. Criminal Justice Involvement 79
22. Estate Planning 80
23. Homelessness 80
24. Ongoing Care & Caregiver Role 81
25. Caregiver Self-care: You Matter Too 84
26. Top 10 Mistakes Caregivers Make 85
27. When You Need More Support 86

PART I:
QUICK START

Identify Your Situation to take Immediate Action

🚨 Immediate Safety Risk

Life-threatening emergency, please call or text 911

If your loved one shows:

☐ Risk of harm to self or others

☐ Suicidal thoughts or behaviors

☐ Loss of control, psychosis, or severe agitation

→ Go to: Part III – Section 6: Crisis & Immediate Safety
→ See also: Part III – Section 8: Suicide Risk & Prevention

Mental Health Crisis
For other mental health crises, please call or text 988
→ Go to: Part III – Section 6: Crisis & Immediate Safety

🚫 Refusing Help

If your loved one shows:

☐ Does not believe anything is wrong

☐ Refuses treatment or support

☐ Conversations escalate into conflict

→ Go to: Part III – Section 10: When They Refuse Help
→ See also: Part II – Section 1: Understanding Bipolar Disorder

⚠ Symptoms Emerging

If your loved one shows:

☐ Reduced need for sleep

☐ Mood or energy changes

☐ Behavior changes

→ Go to: Part III – Section 2: How to Help if Your Loved One Shows Symptoms of Mania or Hypomania
→ See also: Part III – Section 3: How to Help if Your Loved One Shows Symptoms of Depression
→ See also: Part III – Section 5: When Psychosis is Emerging

→ See also: Part III – Section 7: When They Are Not a Danger but Clearly Unwell

💬 Communication or Conflict

If conversations with your loved one:
☐ Escalate quickly
☐ Make you feel uncertain what to say
→ Go to: Part III – Section 11: Reducing Conflict & De-escalation
→ See also: Part III – Section 15: How to Communicate

💊 Treatment Concerns

If you observe the following in your loved one:
☐ Treatment is not working
☐ Side effects or adherence concerns
→ Go to: Part III – Section 9: Screening & Starting Treatment

📊 Monitoring & Prevention

☐ You want to track patterns and early warning signs
→ Go to: Part III – Section 16: Monitoring & Prevention

🌱 Stable/Recovery

If your loved one:
☐ Reached stability
☐ Is focused on long-term recovery
→ Go to: Part III – Section 17: Ready to Pursue Recovery

💔 Caregiver Overwhelmed

If caregiving has made you feel:

☐ You feel burned out

☐ You feel overwhelmed

→ Go to: Part II – Section 11: Peer Support & Community
→ Go to: Part III – Section 25: Caregiver Self-care: You Matter Too
→ See also: Part III – Section 13: Boundaries

PART II:
WHAT TO KNOW

You do not need to read this section. Use it as a reference and return to it when you need deeper understanding.

1. Understanding Bipolar Disorder

Caregivers play an important role in understanding the condition; especially when loved ones are in denial, disengaged, or overwhelmed.

Bipolar disorder:

- Affects moods, behavior, and thinking
- Includes:
  - Mania or hypomania (elevated or irritable, increased energy)
  - Depression (low mood, energy, motivation)
  - Cognitive impairments
- Can include "mixed states," which combines the features of mania and depression
- Is complex and varies widely from person to person
- Has no cure, but can be managed
- Can take time to diagnose; misdiagnosis is common
- Is often initially diagnosed as depression (not bipolar)

There are several types of bipolar disorder:

- The two most common are Bipolar 1 and Bipolar II
- Bipolar I disorder involves episodes of mania
- Bipolar II involves hypomania (a milder form of mania)

Coming to terms with bipolar disorder is often overwhelming. Support from healthcare providers, friends, and family is essential. The first episode is the hardest, but patterns and effective strategies become clearer over time. Learn what helped and what didn't to make future episodes more manageable. And now you'll have a crisis plan in place.

Key Realities

- A common initial reaction to a diagnosis is shock, disbelief, and denial
- Antidepressants for unipolar depression may be prescribed initially (which can trigger mania or hypomania in some cases)
- For most people, depression is the hardest part of bipolar

- People with bipolar disorder often spend significantly more time in depression than in mania or hypomania
- Episodes often develop gradually, allowing time to act before they fully escalate. In other cases, they come on suddenly
- Episodes are recurrent and can last days to months. Tracking may show patterns
- Even after an episode has passed, residual symptoms may persist
- During episodes your loved one may have little to no control over their behavior
- A full, meaningful life is possible (recovery may take time)

Symptoms

Mania

A manic episode typically involves at least a week of elevated or irritable mood, along with increased energy and several additional symptoms. Mania and hypomania can feel enjoyable at first, which may delay help-seeking.

Keep an eye out for the following indicators of a manic episode:

- Decreased need for sleep (feels rested after only a few hours)
- More talkative than usual (rapid, loud, hard to interrupt)
- Racing thoughts or disorganized communication (rapid, loosely connected)
- Easily distracted (attention pulled by minor or irrelevant stimuli)
- Increased irritability (especially when challenged or blocked)
- Increased goal-directed activity (takes on excessive or unrealistic tasks)
- Inflated self-esteem or grandiosity (feels superior, entitled, or unusually talented)
- Impulsive, erratic, or risky behavior (e.g., reckless spending, driving, or sexual behavior)
- Attention-seeking actions that are out of character (e.g., inappropriate social media posts)

Symptoms significantly impair functioning, may require hospitalization, are clearly noticeable to others, and are not caused by substances or medical conditions.

Hypomania

Similar to mania but less severe, lasts at least four days, noticeable to others without causing major impairment or hospitalization, and not due to substances or medication.

See indicators list under Mania above.

Major Depression

Criteria for a major depressive episode:

- Depressed mood or loss of interest
- Causes clear impairment in functioning
- Not due to substances or a medical condition
- Lasts most of the day, nearly every day, for at least two weeks

Keep an eye out for the following indicators of a major depressive episode:

- Loss of interest or pleasure in most activities
- Changes in appetite or weight
- Changes in sleep habits (too little or too much)
- Agitation or slowed movement (noticeable by others)
- Fatigue or low energy
- Feelings of worthlessness or excessive guilt
- Poor concentration or indecisiveness
- Thoughts of death or suicide

Depression can feel permanent, which may intensify hopelessness and, in some cases, contribute to suicidal thinking.

Cognitive Impairments

- Thinking, focus, memory, and decision-making are commonly impaired and can significantly impact daily functioning, decision-making, and independence
- Depending on severity, consider cognitive rehabilitation programs

Psychosis

Delusions = fixed false beliefs. Delusions cannot be reasoned away. Types include:

- Belief conviction: fixed certainty in false beliefs despite clear evidence
- Grandiose (bipolar I): beliefs of exceptional power, wealth, or intelligence
- Guilt (major depression): beliefs of extreme, unwarranted remorse and self-blame

Hallucinations = seeing or hearing things that aren't there; a core feature of psychosis. Types include:

- Auditory (most common): hearing voices, music, or sounds that aren't real
- Visual: seeing people, objects, or lights that aren't there

Post-Manic Depression

Severe depression often follows manic or hypomanic episodes

- Expect a sharp drop in mood, energy, and functioning
- This phase can feel more intense than typical depression, with heightened risk of hopelessness or suicidal thinking

Schizoaffective Disorder, Bipolar Type

Combines features of schizophrenia and bipolar:

- Mood episodes (mania and/or depression)
- Psychotic symptoms (hallucinations or delusions), which can occur even when mood symptoms are not present

Co-occurring Conditions & Symptoms

Bipolar often co-occurs with other conditions, including:

- Anxiety disorders (common)
- Substance use (common)
- Psychosis (particularly in advanced stages of mania)

    - Includes delusions (e.g., grandiosity) and hallucinations
- Anosognosia (lack of insight of illness) is common, especially during mania
    - Your loved one may not believe they are ill

Practical Implications

- Expect complexity: Symptoms may overlap and change over time
- Lack of insight is part of the illness. It is not stubbornness, denial, or unwillingness
    - Arguing or explaining rarely creates insight
    - You may need to act on your loved one's behalf during periods of low insight
- Know that diagnosis is based on:
    - Current behaviors
    - Past history
    - Family history
- Doing what's best for your loved one's recovery can be hard. Hypomania and substance use often increase social activity, and even well-meaning friends can unintentionally impact recovery in some cases

2. Resources & Education

Trusted Resources
- National Alliance on Mental Illness (NAMI)
- Mayo Clinic
- Cleveland Clinic

Lived Experience Resources
Use lived experience resources, which offer insight into what bipolar feels like and what helps:
- bpHope
- International Bipolar Foundation
- Well-known Memoir
    - *An Unquiet Mind* by Kay Redfield Jamison

- Short personal accounts
  - *Psychiatric Services*
  - *Schizophrenia Bulletin*
- Educational Film
  - Brainstorm

3. Types of Hospitalization

Use the least restrictive options whenever possible. Reassure your loved one that your goal is support, not control.

Outpatient Care

- Not admitted (standard care)
- 1–2 appointments per week (therapy and/or medication management)
- Best for mild to moderate symptoms in stable individuals
- Used for ongoing maintenance or step-down from hospitalization

Partial Hospitalization (PHP)

- No immediate safety crisis; not admitted
- Intensive, structured day program: 4–6 hours/day, 4–5 days/week
- Includes psychiatry and multiple therapies (group, individual, skills)
- Close monitoring for serious or worsening symptoms
- Used when weekly care is not enough or to avoid, or as a step down from, hospitalization

Extended ER Observation

In a specialized comprehensive psychiatric emergency program (CPEP)

- Not the same as being admitted to an inpatient unit, but also not being sent home
- Extended evaluation over 1-3 days
- Useful for crisis, uncertainty about whether inpatient care is needed, substance use detox, or when clinicians need more time to decide on best level of care

Voluntary Hospitalization

- Your loved one agrees to self-admit
- Best-case scenario for cooperation and continuity of care
- Returning to the same institution may ease transition; if past experience was unfavorable, consider a fresh start at a different institution

Involuntary Hospitalization

- Criteria: danger to self or others
- Often initiated by caregiver; may generate high conflict
- Last resort for acute crisis
- May include ~72-hour hold for evaluation and treatment
- Can involve medication for agitation, physical restraints, or seclusion
- Rules and procedures vary state-by-state
- Can be both therapeutic and traumatizing; may drastically impact trust and the caregiving relationship

Assisted Outpatient Treatment

- Civil court-ordered outpatient mental health treatment
- Designed for individuals with mental illness who struggle to voluntarily adhere to treatment
- Helps people live and remain successfully in the community
- Aims to reduce repeated hospitalizations, crises, homelessness, or incarceration
- AOT laws vary by state
- A caregiver among others can petition for AOT

4. Insurance

Using Insurance to Find Care

☐ Start with your insurance plan—it will shape your options.

☐ Review your behavioral health coverage

☐ Search your insurance website for in-network providers

Public Insurance (Medicare/Medicaid)

- Government-funded coverage
- Often for low-income individuals, people with disabilities, or older adults
- Fewer providers may accept it
- Medicaid coverage varies by state

☐ Coverage holder should check their Medicare account at Medicare.gov and their state's Medicaid portal (or by calling their customer service lines) to view current enrollment, benefits, and coverage status.

Private Insurance

- Usually provided through an employer or purchased individually

☐ Check in-network vs. out-of-network coverage

Out-of-Network Care

- Some providers do not accept insurance
- You may need to pay upfront

☐ Don't forget to submit claims for possible reimbursement

Tips

☐ Confirm coverage before scheduling

☐ Ask providers directly if they accept your insurance

☐ Clarify costs (copay, deductible, reimbursement)

5. Treatment Team

Prescriber

Psychiatric Nurse Practitioner (NP)

- Can prescribe and manage psychiatric medications
- Often more accessible than psychiatrist and may offer longer visits

Psychiatrist (MD)

- Most extensive training in mental health and medication management

- Treats a wide range of psychiatric conditions
- Bipolar Specialist (if available)
- May have academic or research focus in bipolar, including peer-reviewed publications and active involvement in the bipolar community (e.g., conferences, professional groups)
- Can be harder to find

What to Expect

- Appointments are often brief (e.g., ~15 minutes, medication-focused)

They may also provide therapy or second opinions

Psychopharmacologist

- Psychiatrist with advanced expertise in medication management
- Often focused on complex cases or treatment optimization

Primary Care Provider (PCP)

- Often the first to detect mental health concerns
- Can manage mild to moderate depression or anxiety and refer to a psychiatric specialist when needed

Prescriber – Tips

☐ Ask about experience treating bipolar disorder

☐ Consider a specialist for complex or unclear cases

☐ Combine medication with therapy for best outcomes

Therapists & Other Treatment Specialists

Types of Therapists (also referred to as counselors)

- Licensed Creative Arts Therapists
- Licensed Mental Health Counselors
- Marriage and Family Therapists
- Occupational Therapists
- Pastoral Counselors
- Social Workers
- Psychologists

Case Managers/Care Coordinators

- Clinically trained professionals who help navigate care and systems
- Assist with disability services, housing, and appointment coordination
- Many therapists (especially social workers) also serve in this role
- Routinely assigned for patients on disability but can be privately engaged

Finding the right therapist may take several attempts

☐ Prioritize "fit" as the most important factor, as well as knowledge base

☐ Look for trust, comfort, and strong communication

☐ Respect your loved one's privacy and preferences

Other Treatment Specialists

Certified Peer Specialists (also called peer supporters, navigators, or providers)

Someone with lived experience with serious mental illness, including bipolar who has completed State-approved educational and employment requirements.

- Provides mentorship, support, and practical guidance for recovery
- Often work in public or community mental health settings
- Typically covered by public insurance

Bipolar Coach

Someone with extensive lived experience of bipolar who may also have formal education or professional training.

- Provides mentorship, support, and practical, real-world guidance for recovery
- Typically works privately (outside traditional clinical systems)
- May be difficult to find due to the emerging nature of the profession
- Not typically covered by insurance

Pharmacist
- Monitors for drug–drug interactions and medication safety
- Ensures that psychiatric medications do not conflict with non-psychiatric medication prescribed by other doctors
- Answers questions about medications and adherence

Caregiver
You play a key role as part of the treatment team. Your loved one may struggle to communicate their needs to their providers.

You can help the following ways:
☐ Advocate for your loved one with treatment providers
☐ Do not dismiss concerns about medications or side effects
☐ Recognize that stigma can occur in healthcare settings too. If you observe it, remind healthcare providers that stigma can negatively impact outcomes
☐ Speak up if something does not feel right

6. Medication & Non-Therapy Treatments

Common Medication Types
- Mood stabilizers (e.g., lithium, certain anticonvulsants)
- Antipsychotics (often used for mania; some also used to treat bipolar depression)
- Antidepressants (used cautiously; may be less effective in bipolar than in non-bipolar depression, and can trigger mania)
- Stimulants (used cautiously; typically for co-occurring ADHD)

Medication selection is determined based on symptoms, severity and past treatment response.

Common Side Effects & Management
☐ Remember all medications may potentially cause side effects and require risk benefit discussions
  - Sedation → may improve over time or with adjustments

- Weight gain → manage with diet, exercise, or medication changes

☐ Monitor and report side effects to prescriber early

Serious Side Effects (Watch For)

- Tardive dyskinesia (TD): involuntary movements. Report symptoms immediately as they can be treated; medication decisions should be made with a prescriber.
- Some atypical antipsychotics may cause diabetes and high cholesterol
- Medication decisions should be made with a prescriber.

Other Treatment Options (Treatment-Resistant Depression)

- Ketamine (IV infusion, clinic-based) and esketamine (nasal spray): typically not covered by insurance and costly. Esketamine coverage for bipolar specifically is limited, most plans cover it only for unipolar depression.
- ECT (Electroconvulsive Therapy)
- Bright light therapy
- TMS (Transcranial Magnetic Stimulation)
- Psychedelic-assisted therapy: considered experimental for depression, safety in bipolar is not yet established

Early Intervention for Psychosis

Early identification and treatment can prevent full episodes

☐ Seek care at specialized early intervention programs when possible

☐ Act quickly if early warning signs appear

Treatment Approach

☐ Start with evidence-based or best-practice treatments

☐ Discuss all options openly with your provider

☐ Ask about alternative/complementary treatments (e.g., nutraceuticals, metabolic/ketogenic approaches) and their safety

Medication Coverage

Insurance coverage varies

☐ Verify your benefits

☐ Look for discounts (manufacturer programs, GoodRx, Cost Plus Drugs)

☐ Compare pharmacy prices when possible

7. Therapy Options and Other

General Guidance

- Expect trial and error, finding the right therapist and therapy type may take time
- Be open to trying more than one provider and approach

Talk Therapies That Have Been Shown to be Helpful in Bipolar

- CBT (Cognitive Behavioral Therapy): targets unhelpful thinking patterns and behaviors
- DBT (Dialectical Behavioral Therapy): builds emotion regulation and distress tolerance skills
- FFT (Family-Focused Therapy): includes psychoeducation, communication, and problem-solving skills
- IPSRT (Interpersonal and Social Rhythm Therapy): supports routine, medication adherence, and stability of daily rhythms

Integrated Dual Disorder Treatment

- Mental illness and substance use often occur together and should be treated at the same time since untreated substance use can worsen bipolar symptoms, make treatment less effective, and increase relapse risk.
- Consider providers with expertise in addiction (e.g., addiction psychiatrists)

Note: marijuana use may trigger or worsen psychosis in some individuals

When choosing therapy options, remember to:

☐ Focus on what is most helpful for your loved one's symptoms and needs

☐ Reassess and adjust if progress is limited

☐ Always be person-centered and recovery-oriented

Harm Reduction and Substance Use

- Meet people where they are; any positive change counts
- Ask them to never use alone; keep naloxone on hand
- Know overdose signs; call 911
- Encourage safer choices: avoid mixing substances
- Consider safety tools such as naloxone, fentanyl test strips; use sterile equipment
- Connect to resources, not ultimatums
- Harm reduction does not mean approval. It means reducing danger and keeping the door open to treatment

8. Community-Based Services

Certified Community Behavioral Health Centers (CCBHCs)

- Federally certified by the Department of Health & Human Services
- Located throughout the U.S.
- Provide services regardless of ability to pay

Services Offered

- 24/7 crisis services
- Comprehensive behavioral health care
- Care coordination across systems (mental health, physical health, social services)

Access

☐ Use findtreatment.gov to locate a center near you

Mobile Crisis Unit

- Community-based programs that bring a mental health professional into the home to evaluate mental health needs, assess potential need for hospital evaluation, and identify how to make better use of outpatient resources
- You can find them by calling your local 211 information line. It's a step before calling 911.

Assertive Community Treatment (ACT)

- Team-based, "whole-person" approach to care
- Provides services in the community (not just clinic-based)
- Services include:
    - Mental health treatment
    - Integrated treatment for substance use (dual diagnosis)
    - Family education and support
    - Peer support
    - Community integration support
    - Vocational/employment support

Access

- Designed for individuals with more complex or severe needs

☐ Ask providers or CCBHCs about referrals to ACT programs

9. Psychoeducation

☐ Learn about the condition (symptoms, course, and treatment)

☐ Identify personal triggers and early warning signs

☐ Develop coping strategies to manage symptoms; identify factors that may interfere with their effectiveness and ways to minimize interference

10. Health Risks & Monitoring

- Bipolar is associated with reduced life expectancy most often due to undertreated medical problems such as heart disease, obesity, smoking/emphysema

- Monitor for common conditions (thyroid disorders, diabetes, cardiovascular disease, kidney disease, COPD, chronic pain)
- Address lifestyle risk factors, especially tobacco use
- Even with good treatment episodes may still occur; but their impact can be reduced, quality of life improved, and the frequency of episodes may decrease.

11. Peer Support & Community

Peer support is invaluable and it's being used more and more because it works. It can help both people with mental illness and caregivers.

Benefits of Peer Support

Connection & Understanding
- Reduces isolation and connects you with people who "get it"
- Provides validation through shared lived experience
- Helps normalize symptoms and struggles

Hope & Motivation
- Increases hope by seeing others in recovery
- Reinforces that a meaningful life is possible
- Encourages persistence during setbacks

Practical Guidance
- Offers real-world coping strategies that have worked for others
- Shares insights on navigating treatment, providers, and systems
- Helps problem-solve everyday challenges

Engagement in Care
- Improves willingness to seek and stay in treatment
- Builds trust in the recovery process
- Supports medication adherence and follow-through

Identity & Self-Worth
- Reduces self-stigma and shame

- Strengthens sense of identity beyond the illness
- Helps individuals feel less like a “patient” and more like a person

Emotional Support
- Provides a safe space to share openly
- Offers empathy without judgment
- Helps regulate emotions through connection

Independence & Empowerment
- Encourages self-advocacy and autonomy
- Supports confidence in managing one’s condition
- Promotes recovery-oriented thinking (not just symptom control)

Types of Peer Support

- Certified Peer Specialists (CPSs): individuals with lived experience who provide guidance and support
    - Where to find them? CPSs often work at certified community behavioral health centers (CCBHCs)
- Bipolar Coaches: individuals with lived experience who provide practical, real-world guidance
    - Where to find them? Requires online research and potential referrals
- Warmlines warmline.org: peer-run phone lines offering emotional support (often through CCBHCs)
- Clubhouses (e.g., Fountain House): community spaces focused on relationships, wellness, education, and employment
- NAMI programs: peer-to-peer and family-to-family classes and peer support groups
  DBSA (Depression and Bipolar Support Alliance): peer support groups
- Support groups that focus primarily on problems can sometimes feel discouraging or overwhelming.

12. Emotional Support Animals (ESAs)

Many people find emotional support animals helpful

- Many types of animals can provide emotional support, especially dogs
- Can encourage routine, activity, and exercise
- May reduce loneliness and provide comfort
- For a pet to be considered an ESA legally, you must have a prescription letter from a licensed therapist or doctor. Such a letter may be required for housing related accommodations where pets are not permitted

☐ Ensure your loved one can reliably care for the animal:

  ☐ Assess ability during both stable and symptomatic periods

  ☐ Have a backup plan for care if needed

13. Privacy & Legal (HIPAA)

Consent & Access

Providers need your loved one's consent to share information (Health Insurance Portability and Accountability Act - HIPAA)

- Caregivers must exercise care about what and when important information (e.g., non-adherence, substance use, poor functioning) gets communicated to the provider
- You may have to risk alienating your loved one if they are headed for trouble and unwilling to permit you to step in. It's extremely important, because one of the most valuable roles a caregiver can play is offering the treatment team a clear, accurate picture of what's happening

☐ Discuss and obtain consent when your loved one is stable

☐ Ask your loved one to list you as an emergency contact

Planning Ahead

☐ Put permissions in place before a crisis occurs

☐ Clarify what information can be shared and with whom

☐ Keep documentation accessible if needed

Communication with Providers

- You can share concerns with providers at any time
- Providers cannot share specific information with you without consent
- Providers can share general (not specific to patient) information about the condition and treatment

Caregiver Considerations

☐ Be proactive about obtaining permission to receive information regarding your loved one's medical care - lack of consent can limit involvement during crises

☐ Revisit permissions periodically as circumstances change

14. Government Benefits (think long term)

Mindset

When considering applying for government benefits:

☐ Remember that this support is not necessarily permanent

☐ Recognize that a work disruption may be necessary to address your loved one's mental health. Benefits can provide critical financial and healthcare support.

☐ Avoid assuming your loved one cannot work again

☐ Keep future potential and goals in mind

☐ Try to balance following objectives:

  ☐ Support both stability and purpose

  ☐ Prioritize financial security while maintaining identity, goals, and meaning

Key Benefits

- SSI (Supplemental Security Income)
- SSDI (Social Security Disability Insurance)
- Medicaid and Medicare
- Veterans Affairs (VA) benefits
- SNAP (food assistance)

- Public housing programs

Verify current rules with a benefits counselor or attorney, as these change

Application & Support

☐ Recognize the application process can be complex

☐ Seek help from community organizations (e.g., CCBHCs, Clubhouses)

ABLE Account

☐ Consider an ABLE account (tax-advantaged savings for disabilities)

- Allows saving money without affecting SSI eligibility
- Can be used for approved expenses

Ticket to Work Program

How It Helps

- Fear of losing government-sponsored benefits (especially health insurance) often prevents return to work
- Allows individuals to work and earn income up to certain limits while maintaining certain benefits, including healthcare coverage
- Provides a pathway to gradually re-enter the workforce
- Offers support services for employment
- Rules may vary state-to-state

Important Considerations

☐ Carefully review your loved one's government benefits as rules and limits can be complex and vary by program

☐ Verify how work may impact SSI, SSDI, and healthcare coverage

☐ Seek guidance from benefits counselors or community organizations. Consider working with a benefits specialist to navigate eligibility, applications, and potential impacts. You may be able to find them at CCBHCs.

PART III:
WHAT TO DO

Use this section to identify specific actions to take or consider based on your loved one's current condition. While it may be useful to read the following in order, it is not necessary. You can jump to specific sections that best relate to what you and your loved one are experiencing.

1. Understanding their Experience

Understanding how your loved one may be feeling can help you respond more effectively, and with greater empathy.

They May be Feeling

- Misunderstood
- Fear (relapse, consequences, loss of control)
- Shame (especially after episodes)
- Frustration (with illness or treatment)
- Grief (lost time, identity, opportunities)
- Failure
- Hope (especially in recovery)

Toward You, They May Feel

- Like a burden
- That they've disappointed you
- Fear of abandonment
- Unloved or unlovable
- That you are overreacting

Important Reminders

- Each person is different
- Stigma is powerful, do not underestimate it.
- Caregivers and their loved ones need a shared understanding of bipolar
- Experience will guide you
- Help your loved one maintain a sense of control and agency
- Stability may be the immediate goal but recovery is the destination
- Recovery means a full, meaningful life, however your loved one defines it

Lack of Understanding Can Contribute to:

- Conflict and hurtful interactions (e.g., "I hate you")
- Withdrawal or loss of communication

- Refusal of help or treatment
- Worsening symptoms
- Substance use
- Self-destructive behavior
- Family instability
- Legal or housing consequences

Many caregivers underestimate how quickly things can spiral.

Bipolar disorder can be devastating but it is manageable.

☐ Learn the symptoms → See Part II – Section 1

☐ Identify effective coping strategies → See Part III – Section 2

☐ Learn to recognize early warning signs of mood changes → See Part III – Section 16

☐ Know how and where to get help from providers, crisis resources, support systems → See Part III

2. How To Help if Your Loved One Shows Symptoms of Mania or Hypomania

Immediate Actions:

☐ Check crisis plan → See Part III – Section 14
☐ Be patient
☐ Stay calm and grounded, don't match their intensity
☐ Validate without reinforcing behavior
☐ Reduce stimulation (noise, activity, and social contact)
☐ Prioritize their sleep, encourage rest
☐ Stay close without being controlling
☐ Delay major decisions (spending, travel, commitments)
☐ Encourage professional care
☐ Involve trusted supports
☐ Gently but firmly ask your loved one if they have been missing medication doses.
- If you suspect your loved one may not be fully adherent, it can be difficult to raise this with them, but this is important information to obtain
- The most common reason for relapse is not taking medications properly

☐ Recognize certain symptoms stand out for their severity (e.g., suicidal thoughts or behaviors and psychotic features)
☐ Consider need to modify environment
☐ Share helpful information through calm conversation or by offering resources to read. This can reduce confrontation, especially during agitation

If your loved one has previously had a manic episode:
☐ Recognize that no single symptom automatically equates to relapse; instead look for collections or constellations of symptoms

☐ Distinguish persistence of symptoms from blips (brief or fleeting symptoms that do not evolve into full episodes and may not require intervention) and patterns

Recognize that the conversation may not be productive in the moment:

☐ Do not try to interrupt or compete

☐ Revisit important topics later

☐ Wait until they are calmer and more able to engage:

- Avoid trying to reason or debate
- Look for natural pauses before speaking
- Gently redirect if needed
- Keep it simple and non-confrontational
- Focus on listening, not correcting
- Use reality testing (gently question beliefs without confrontation)

☐ Acknowledge that hypomania can feel enticing but that it can worsen their condition

Stabilization

☐ Implement risk-reduction strategies (limit risk, delay decisions)

☐ Set gentle limits on risky behavior

☐ Protect finances and safety if necessary (e.g., securing credit cards and car keys)

☐ Apply de-escalation techniques (below)

Communication

☐ Use brief, clear communication

☐ Do not argue or confront

☐ Do not tell them they are "sick" in the moment

☐ Avoid language that feels controlling or critical

☐ Focus on common ground and assuring everyone's safety. Defer emotionally charged conversations to quieter times

3. How to Help if Your Loved One Shows Symptoms of Depression

Higher Risk—Act Immediately

If your loved one exhibits following behaviors:

☐ Talking about death or being a burden
☐ Significant withdrawal or isolation
☐ Giving away possessions or saying goodbye
☐ Sudden worsening or abrupt mood shift

→ Go to: Part III – Section 6: Crisis & Immediate Safety
→ See also: Part III – Section 8: Suicide Risk & Prevention

Use the Following Communication Strategies:

☐ Be present, do not try to fix
☐ Listen without interrupting
☐ Validate distress
☐ Use reframing to counter negative self-talk
☐ Check in consistently
☐ Encourage one trusted connection
☐ Encourage professional care
☐ Offer practical support (meals, errands, scheduling and providing transportation to healthcare appointments)
☐ Support basic functioning (sleep, meals, hygiene)
☐ Maintain simple structure
☐ Reduce demands, focus on essentials only
☐ Ask direct, simple questions, avoid overwhelming
☐ See if they will respond to offers of distraction (if unable to may reflect greater severity)
☐ Encourage activity (even small steps)

☐ Keep a list of activities for every mood, the most effective ones involve physical activity, take place outdoors, and are shared with friends or family.
☐ Staying active can help reduce rumination on negative thoughts, which are common and may otherwise worsen depression.
☐ Don't let them stay in bed all day
☐ Encourage the use of coping skills such as journaling
☐ Avoid labeling them as lazy (lack of motivation is a symptom known as "avolition") and instead use gentle nudges to promote physical activity
☐ Provide extra support and monitoring in periods of post-manic depression
☐ If they are crying just maintain a non-judgmental presence, offer comfort (water, tissues) and remain present unless they ask for space, and ask them if they know how you can be helpful

Avoid
☐ Minimizing (e.g., "just stay positive", "it can't be that bad")
☐ Arguing or challenging feelings
☐ Taking control
☐ Withdrawing or waiting for them to reach out
☐ Accusing a loved one of "making up their symptoms" can create significant conflict and may discourage them from reaching out to you.

When Post-Manic Depression is Emerging:
☐ Recognize early signs (withdrawal, low energy, hopelessness)
☐ Take changes in mood or behavior seriously
☐ Stay present, even quiet presence helps
☐ Keep communication simple and low pressure
☐ Avoid trying to "fix" or solve the depression
☐ Avoid statements like "just think positive" or "snap out of it"
☐ Validate their experience ("I'm here with you")
☐ Help them feel needed, ask for small forms of help, like easy chores

☐ Expect low motivation (avolition), do not interpret as laziness

Support in the Moment

☐ Offer small, manageable steps (eat, shower, short walk)
☐ Help break tasks into small actions or steps
☐ Offer to do things with them, not for them
☐ Gently encourage routine (sleep, meals, basic structure)
☐ Simplify choices and expectations so your loved one is not overwhelmed
☐ Protect energy, limit unnecessary demands

Stabilization

☐ Focus on getting through the day, not solving everything
☐ Maintain basic structure (sleep, food, medications)
☐ Encourage connection (text, brief visit, low effort contact)
☐ Support adherence to treatment plan
☐ Ask the prescriber about medication adjustments if symptoms worsen, and whether as-needed medication can be kept on hand for early symptoms

Safety

☐ Take any talk of hopelessness or death seriously
☐ Ask directly about suicidal thoughts if concerned (e.g., "are you having any thoughts about wanting to hurt yourself or wanting to be dead." If they answer yes, there needs to be a management/crisis plan. See Crisis Plan Part III, section 14.
☐ Do not leave them alone if risk is elevated
☐ Contact supports (provider, crisis line) if needed

Communication

☐ Keep language simple, calm, and non-judgmental
☐ Avoid minimizing or comparing ("others have it worse")
☐ Avoid pressure, urgency, or frustration
☐ Repeat support consistently ("I'm here")

4. When Cognitive Impairments are Emerging

☐ Discuss cognitive impairments with provider.
☐ Consider emergency evaluation if your loved one is grossly cognitively impaired, (e.g., unable to follow instructions, confused, disoriented)

5. When Psychosis is Emerging

☐ Consider that psychosis may be present if your loved one presents a rigidly inflexible stance or belief about a position
☐ Carefully follow communication strategies provided here
☐ Do not argue or debate ("That's not true")
☐ Do not try to prove them wrong with facts or logic
☐ Reaffirm whether medications are being taken consistently
☐ Consider whether an extra or as needed dose has been ordered for as needed use
☐ If psychosis is a new symptom, it needs evaluation. Notify prescriber.

6. Crisis & Immediate Safety

If there is any concern about safety, treat it as a crisis. It's always better to act early. Crisis can include agitation, potential for violent behavior, acute intoxication, suicidality, self-harm, sudden change in thinking pattern.

☐ Act immediately

☐ **Call or text 911** when there is an **immediate threat to life or safety** to the person experiencing the crisis

- Dispatches emergency responders to callers' location and may provide support to the caller while waiting for services to arrive
- Emergency responders may include EMTs, police or fire teams
- Emergency responders may proceed with evaluation or involuntary hospitalization
- Have someone stay with loved one while someone else calls 911, if possible

☐ **Call or text 988 or chat 988lifeline.org** when there is **no immediate danger posed** to the person experiencing the crisis or others

- Provides someone experiencing a mental health crisis or emotional distress someone with training to talk to
- Trained crisis counselors provide support, assess risk, help de-escalate the situation, and connect to support services

☐ Stay with person experience the crisis if safe

☐ Prioritize safety—including your own

  ☐ Remove or secure means of harm

☐ Stay calm

☐ Expect anger—don't take it personally (this will be extremely hard)

☐ Remind yourself you are acting out of care and love

☐ Reach out to clinician for guidance

911 or 988 A Quick Guide

When someone is in emotional distress or experiencing a mental health crisis, it can be difficult to know whether to call 988 or 911

Call 911 when any of the below is happening:

□ A suicide attempt is occurring or has just occurred

□ There is an immediate danger to life or safety. These situations may include when the person experiencing the mental health crisis:

- □ Has a weapon or has made a violent threat
- □ Is physically harming themselves or someone else
- □ Is unconscious, severely injured, overdosing, or medically unstable

Call, text or chat 988 helpline when any of the below is happening:

□ **There is no immediate physical danger** but the person experiencing the mental health crisis:

- □ Is having thoughts or feelings of suicide but is not actively attempting suicide
- □ Is experiencing severe depression, anxiety, panic, or emotional distress
- □ Is overwhelmed and needs immediate mental health support
- □ Is agitated or behaving unusually but is not threatening harm to themselves or others

□ Your loved one is experiencing emotional distress and just needs someone to talk to

□ You need guidance about how to respond to a mental health crisis

□ You need support for substance use problems

If You Are Unsure

□ Start with 988 if there is no immediate physical danger.

□ Call 911 immediately if the situation becomes life-threatening or unsafe

□ When safety is in question, err on the side of caution

Remember: You do not have to manage a crisis alone. Seeking help early can prevent a situation from escalating.

Other Support

- Crisis Text Line text HOME to 741741
- Local Mobile Crisis Services/Crisis Intervention Teams (search local crisis team)
- Disaster Distress Helpline 1-800-985-5990
- Trevor Project (for LGBTQ+ youth) 1-866-488-7386, text 678678
- US Veterans Crisis Line Dial 988 then press 1, text 838255

7. When They Are Not a Danger but Clearly Unwell

Unwell means any of the following are true about your loved one's condition:

☐ Their condition is interfering with work, relationships, or self-care (e.g., hygiene, eating and drinking, sleep)?
☐ Their symptoms are intense, escalating, or hard to manage?
☐ Their symptoms have persisted or worsened over time?

If your loved one is not in crisis but is unwell:

☐ Act quickly
- Early action can prevent worsening condition
- Do not delay: Delays can make treatment more difficult

☐ Consider hospitalization for immediate treatment
  ☐ See below and Part II – Section 3: Types of Hospitalization
☐ If your loved one has a substance use or personality disorder, consider a residential treatment facility – See below for more information
☐ Seek support and guidance from helplines – See below for more information

Choosing Hospital Care

Most hospitalizations occur through ER following a 911 call. The choice of hospitalization will depend on local resource availability and possibly insurance restrictions. If your loved one is not in crisis, you can help research and find the best hospital option:

☐ Research top psychiatric hospitals (e.g., U.S. News & World Report rankings)
☐ Consider teaching hospitals (often more specialized programs)

Certain hospitals have national reputations for planned, elective non-emergency admissions for more comprehensive diagnostic and treatment evaluations (e.g., McLean Hospital in Belmont, MA or Menninger Clinic in Dallas, TX), which are often self-pay.

What to Expect from Hospitalization

- Length of stay is typically short (i.e., less than a week)
- Goal is crisis stabilization and transition to outpatient care
- Contact time with doctors is often limited; more extensive time spent in groups
- Evaluations are less comprehensive than those in outpatient settings, but provide a safer environment when self-harm and harm to others is a risk
- Certain treatments, such as ECT, are often begun inpatient
- Electronic devices are often not permitted
- The inpatient team ideally communicates with the outpatient treatment provider to coordinate care and aftercare
- The social worker on the team will customarily reach out to the caregiver to proactively schedule a family meeting

Hospital Visits

☐ Visit as often as possible unless the hospital staff advises against, even if your loved one:

- Seems unaware
- Is angry or resistant

☐ If your loved one requests no visitors, use your judgment and consult staff as needed, since preferences and needs may change during a crisis

☐ Do not be surprised if staff:

  - Prohibits or limits visits they believe may be counterproductive
  - Requires supervised visits

☐ Bring comfort items:

  - Favorite foods (if allowed)
  - Comfortable clothes
  - Simple activities that may help them pass the time

Discharge Planning (critical)

☐ Ensure a transition and discharge plan is in place before leaving

☐ Do not assume the hospital has communicated with your outpatient treatment provider

☐ Establish a follow-up plan for:

- Psychiatric appointments
- Therapy
- Medications
- Housing/living arrangements

☐ Ensure your loved one's belongings, including any of their personal medication they brought, are returned at discharge

☐ Know what to do if symptoms worsen after discharge (e.g., return to hospital or call your doctor)

Residential Treatment Facilities

- Residential treatment facilities (e.g., Gould Farm), which are often useful for

chronic conditions such as substance use and personality disorders

☐ Consider sober living facilities for a longer-term therapeutic environment for your loved ones with substance use disorders

☐ Check with insurance, as many residential programs require full or partial self-pay

☐ Ask your treatment providers for referrals

Helplines

☐ Use helplines for guidance (not crisis)

☐ Contact the NAMI Helpline

- Call 1-800-950-NAMI (6264)
- Text "Helpline" to 62640

☐ Explore local NAMI resources

- Many affiliates offer local helplines and support

8. Suicide Risk & Prevention

Bipolar disorder carries elevated suicide risk

☐ Learn key risk factors, protective factors, and warning signs from the American Foundation for Suicide Prevention website

☐ Identify high-risk situations in advance:

  ☐ Note any prior suicide attempts, and be particularly vigilant if one has occurred

  ☐ Assess access to lethal means (e.g., firearms, excess medication) and eliminate access where possible

Screening (ask directly)

☐ Ask Suicide-Screening Questions (ASQ), such as

- In the past few weeks, have you wished you were dead?
- In the past few weeks, have you felt that you or your family would be better off if you were dead?
- In the past week, have you been having thoughts about killing yourself?
- Have you ever tried to kill yourself?
- Are you having thoughts of killing yourself right now?

☐ Do not avoid the topic; talking about suicide does NOT increase risk

Prevention & Awareness

☐ Identify triggers of suicidal thoughts and behaviors, which are often linked to mood episodes, stress, or sleep disruption

☐ Monitor changes closely, such as:

- Withdrawal
- Hopelessness
- Sudden shifts in mood

If You're Concerned Trust Your Instincts

☐ Do not wait, act immediately

☐ Contact 988 or emergency services if needed

☐ Intervene decisively, even if they object

9. Screening & Starting Treatment

Screening

☐ Use a screening tool, such as the Mental Health America Bipolar Screening Tool, to assess symptoms

☐ Use results to help determine whether to seek treatment

☐ Know that only a qualified provider can make a formal diagnosis

Rule Out Medical Causes

☐ Start with a primary care provider (PCP) to rule out non-psychiatric causes

☐ Ask your PCP to check for thyroid issues, vitamin deficiencies, infections (e.g., Lyme disease), and other medical conditions

☐ Keep in mind that substance use can mimic the symptoms of mood disorder and requires its own treatment

Learn About Insurance Options

☐ See Part II – Section 4

Learn About Different Types of Providers & Treatments

☐ See Part II – Sections 5 and 6

Starting Treatment

☐ Create a treatment plan to stay organized and in control

☐ Start with a psychiatrist, as medication can provide faster symptom relief

☐ If stigma is a barrier for your loved one, consider starting with a primary care provider (PCP), but keep in mind that many PCPs have limited familiarity with bipolar disorder

☐ Work with a therapist, who can help with:

- Assessment and support
- Transition to psychiatric care

Build the Right Treatment Team

☐ Prioritize finding best-fit providers

  ☐ Look for providers who focus on quality of life, not just symptom reduction

  ☐ See "Ask Your Loved One and Yourself (Provider-Patient Fit) and "Watch For (Poor Fit)" below

☐ Combine medication and therapy when possible (best outcomes)

☐ Consider a prescriber early for symptom relief, and/or when symptoms are severe

☐ Consider an integrated care team (mental + physical health)

☐ Help coordinate care between providers when possible

☐ Develop an understanding of the roles of each member of the treatment team

  ☐ Ask each member of the treatment team to clarify their role so you know who to contact about a certain problem

☐ Ask yourself if you know when to contact the therapist or the prescriber

If Something Isn't Working

☐ Reassess provider fit if concerns arise

☐ Distinguish between

- Discomfort with feedback (part of growth)
- Poor fit (not the right provider)

☐ Find a second opinion or new provider if needed

Where to Find Treatment Team Members

☐ Search your insurance company's directory for in-network providers

☐ Ask friends and family for referrals

☐ Request a referral from your loved one's primary care provider (PCP), therapist, or prescriber; team members who know each other tend to collaborate more effectively

☐ Use online therapist directories, keeping in mind that some require providers to pay to be listed

☐ Review multiple sources to find the best fit

What to Bring to Initial Appointment?

☐ Medical history (including past and current medications and lab records)
☐ Family mental health history (if known)
☐ List of symptoms/behaviors and how they depart from normal
☐ Timeline of when symptoms occurred and how long they lasted
☐ Notes on severity, triggers, or patterns (if known)
☐ Notes on impairments to functioning
☐ Your own file of a copy of pertinent records

What to Ask Prospective Treatment Providers (Initial Appointment)

☐ Approach: Do they focus only on symptom reduction or also on quality of life and recovery?
☐ Insurance: Do they accept your insurance?
☐ Education & Training: Where did they complete their training, and how do they stay current with new developments?
☐ Certifications: Do they hold relevant specialty certifications?
☐ Areas of Expertise: Is their experience relevant to your needs (e.g., bipolar disorder)?
☐ Academic Affiliation: Are they involved in teaching or research?
☐ Publications: Have they published peer-reviewed works, books, or other media?
☐ Availability: Is the provider accessible in terms of appointment frequency, responsiveness, and in the case of emergencies?
☐ Practical Fit:
    ☐ Does the provider work with your insurance?
    ☐ Are cost, location, telehealth options manageable?

Ask Your Loved One and Yourself (Provider-Patient Fit)

☐ Feeling Heard: Does your loved one feel heard, respected, and taken seriously?

☐ Communication Style: Does the provider listen without interrupting or dismissing concerns, explain things clearly, and avoid being rushed or overly technical?

☐ Openness: Does your loved one feel comfortable asking questions and speaking openly?

☐ Collaboration: Is the provider willing to involve your loved one in decisions while respecting their autonomy?

☐ Experience:

- ☐ Are you comfortable with their level of experience, particularly with your specific condition?
- ☐ Does the provider seem comfortable managing the level of complexity (mild vs. severe, comorbidities) of your loved ones disorder?

☐ Trust and Clarity:

- ☐ Does your loved one leave appointments feeling clearer and safer, not more confused or dismissed?
- ☐ Does clinician provide a detailed and thorough evaluation?
- ☐ Does your loved one feel they receive clear instructions and guidance from their provider? If not, ask if the provider will provide written instructions especially when they are complex or easy to forget.

Watch For (Signs of Poor Fit)

☐ Your loved one feels rushed, judged, or not believed

☐ Concerns are minimized or ignored

☐ One-size-fits-all approach with little personalization

☐ Poor communication or lack of follow-up

Working with Providers

☐ Listen carefully to your loved one's concerns about their provider

☐ Take concerns seriously and explore whether the issue is provider fit or discomfort with feedback; don't automatically assume a different clinician would be a better choice if your loved one is rejecting sound advice

☐ Ask whether they feel heard, respected, and understood

☐ If a better fit is needed, look for a new provider but do not stop care until one is in place

☐ Advocate for your loved one and encourage self-advocacy, keeping in mind that:

- Working with providers can feel intimidating
- Stigma in healthcare settings can occur, so you may need to speak up if needed

Shared Decision-Making Approach

☐ Uses an empowering, collaborative approach to treatment

☐ Encourages open communication and builds trust

☐ Supports better adherence to the treatment plan

☐ Your loved one is encouraged to express concerns and preferences

☐ Provider clearly presents and explains treatment options

☐ Provider asks if you have any questions and invites your input

☐ Your loved one and provider discuss options together

☐ Decisions are made collaboratively—not imposed

☐ Your loved one has a meaningful role in choosing the treatment plan

Medication & Other Treatment

☐ Emphasize quality-of-life benefits (e.g., ability to work, function)

☐ Most people with bipolar take medication (often more than one)

☐ Expect trial and error, multiple trials and different medications may be needed

☐ Allow time for medications to take effect

☐ Ask about common side effects and how to manage them if they occur

☐ Ensure your prescriber is open to discussing medications

☐ Know what to expect from each medication

☐ See Part II - Section 6: Medication and Other Treatments

Medication Adherence

Non-adherence is common and a leading cause of relapse. Common barriers include stigma and side effects.

☐ Do not stop or change medication without speaking to your prescriber

☐ Address issues early: options may include dose changes, switching, or adding medications to manage side effects

☐ Know that stopping medication when feeling better is common and can significantly increase relapse risk; some people may also feel that medication is holding them back

☐ Ask whether a long-acting injectable may be appropriate. Since not administered daily, injectables can help with longer-term compliance

☐ Avoid repeatedly asking whether your loved one has taken their medication, as this can be intrusive and may cause them to shut you out of their treatment

☐ If you suspect your loved one is not taking their medication, gently express concern; focus on genuine care for their well-being rather than accusations or ultimatums

Additional Risks

☐ Watch for self-medication (e.g., alcohol or substance use)

☐ Be aware of risk for dual diagnosis (mental health + substance use)

☐ Seek support early if concerns arise

☐ Consider small incentives or rewards, like getting their favorite meal, early on to support medication adherence

Advocacy

☐ Advocate for your loved one's best person-centered, recovery-oriented care

☐ Encourage your loved one to advocate for themselves

☐ Stay engaged, as active participation can improve outcomes

☐ Prioritize helping your loved one build their own self-advocacy skills

☐ Consider encouraging your loved one to meet with a peer support counselor

Prevention & Maintenance

☐ Stay up to date on routine medical care and screenings

☐ Prioritize sleep, nutrition, exercise, and overall wellness

10. When They Refuse Help

Refusing help is common and your response matters. Refusing help is commonly refusing medication or other treatment. It may also involve refusing to follow recommended lifestyle changes such as abstaining from alcohol and substances and other self-care.

☐ First: reduce resistance

- Stay calm and avoid power struggles
- Acknowledge their perspective
- Focus on their goals, not the diagnosis
- Offer choices, not ultimatums
- Lower the barrier, start small
- Time conversations for moments when they are calm

☐ Keep the relationship strong

- Set respectful boundaries
- Protect the relationship, connection matters more than being "right"
- Keep the door open-even if they say no
- Expect this to take time

☐ Understand what may be driving your loved one's refusal, which may include:

  - Not being ready for change (e.g., not wanting to give up an addiction)
  - Stigma or fear
  - Fear of hospitalization or loss of control
  - Negative past experiences or concerns about side effects
  - Lack of insight (anosognosia)
  - Feeling blamed or judged
  - Lack of motivation or apathy

What Helps (strategy)

☐ Use a collaborative approach (work with them, not on them)

☐ Emphasize quality of life (sleep, stress, relationships)
☐ Normalize help-seeking
☐ Involve trusted people (with permission)

Set Expectations (important)

☐ Be clear about possible consequences of refusing help:

- Symptoms may worsen and become harder to treat
- Risk of crisis or hospitalization
- Loss of functioning or independence

When to Shift Approach

☐ If safety is at risk: act immediately (call 988 or 911)
☐ If functioning is declining: act sooner rather than later

Mindset for Caregivers

- You cannot force insight or readiness
- Your influence comes from trust, not control
- Small shifts matter

Increasing Acceptance of Help

☐ Frame it as their decision and avoid pressure; offer choices instead of ultimatums
☐ Emphasize personal benefits (e.g., improved work, relationships, independence)
☐ Focus on quality of life, not just symptoms or diagnosis
☐ Keep initial steps simple and low-effort, especially when they are depressed (e.g., telehealth, flexible timing, minimal barriers)
☐ Reassure them that their privacy will be respected and that they will retain control over who is informed
☐ Reduce fear by clarifying what to expect and addressing concerns about hospitalization
☐ Use respectful boundaries when needed (e.g., "I'm here to support you, but I can't continue X if things don't change")
☐ Start with small, manageable first steps
☐ Consider offering incentives for adherence

11. Reducing Conflict & De-escalation

Anger and irritability are common symptoms. While not acceptable, understanding them can help you respond more effectively.

Minimize Conflict

☐ Prioritize reducing arguments, as conflict can trigger or worsen symptoms

☐ Focus on prevention; catch misunderstandings early before they escalate

☐ Stay aware of your influence; you can often de-escalate or redirect the situation

☐ Accept that not everything is in your control and that some conflict is unavoidable

☐ Use de-escalation strategies consistently, such as

- Maintaining a calm tone
- Pausing and creating space
- Setting clear boundaries

☐ Consider working with a therapist to build communication and de-escalation skills

De-escalation Techniques

☐ Do not take anger personally; it is often driven by the illness, not you

☐ Move to a private, low-stimulation space and limit public exposure

☐ Offer appropriate validation to help reduce escalation

☐ Take a cooling-off period; pause the conversation if emotions escalate

☐ Show empathy and avoid judgment

☐ Respect personal boundaries, keeping in mind that fear of losing control may limit what your loved one feels comfortable sharing

☐ Avoid overreacting, even when it is difficult

☐ Do not engage with challenging or provocative questions

☐ Set clear, simple boundaries and allow silence

☐ Give space for emotions to settle and allow time for decisions; do not rush or pressure
☐ Prioritize safety; leave if the situation becomes unsafe
☐ Encourage your loved one to use a mindfulness app when symptoms emerge (e.g., Insight Timer, Headspace, Calm)

12. What To Do After a Crisis

☐ Learn from the experience: identify what helped and what didn't
☐ Reassure your loved one:

- Emphasize that things can go better next time
- Let your loved one guide the conversation
- Help them understand their behavior occurred when they were ill
- Reduce shame and embarrassment where possible
- Reassure them they deserve healthy, supportive relationships
- Challenge negative self-beliefs (e.g., "I'm a burden/failure/unlovable")

☐ Acknowledge the difficult dynamics of the crisis:

- Apologize for difficult decisions, but don't expect forgiveness
- Offer forgiveness
- Be clear that certain behaviors were not acceptable, while recognizing that impaired inhibition is a common symptom of bipolar disorder

☐ Set clear expectations and boundaries, for example:

- Limit access to finances during reckless periods
- Tie support to treatment adherence

☐ Be thoughtful about discussing past episodes (sometimes it's better not to revisit the details)
☐ Focus on positive change going forward rather than revising details of prior incidents
☐ Prepare for the next crisis by creating or updating a crisis plan (e.g., a PAD) while your loved one is stable

13. Boundaries

There are many situations where a crisis can arise due to harmful or risky behavior.
Setting boundaries or conditions, such as "house rules", can help caregivers protect safety, stability, and their own well-being while still being compassionate. Examples include:

- Restricting access to financial resources or vehicles
- House rules such:
    - Refraining from substance use
    - Expectations for a daily schedule, such as personal hygiene

Key Principles

- Imposing boundaries is a sign that you care
- Boundaries are a protection, not punishment but your loved one may experience them that way
- Boundaries must be clear, stated calmly, and consistently enforced
- It is important to follow through on set boundaries
- Expect pushback at first. This does not mean the boundary is wrong
- The goal is safety and long-term recovery, not short-term comfort

Consider Incentives First (When Appropriate)

☐ Before setting a boundary, consider offering positive incentives for healthy behavior. It may feel like a bribe, but it can be an effective intervention for example:

- "If you take your medication as agreed, I will support X and provide a weekly allowance of $___."
- "If you allow me to speak to your prescriber or therapist, I will support X and provide a weekly allowance of $___."

Examples of Boundaries

Treatment

- "I will only help you pay for school if you get help."
- "I will help with your bills if you adhere to treatment."

- "If you stop medication and become unsafe, I will contact your prescriber."

Substance Use

- "I will not allow drugs or alcohol in the home."
- "If substance use continues, we will need to change our living arrangement."

Harmful or Risky Behavior

- "I won't provide money that could be used for harmful behavior."
- "I will help with essentials (food, housing), but not unrestricted cash."
- "You are welcome to stay here if basic rules are followed (no violence, no substances)."
- "If these rules are broken, there will be consequences."
- "If I believe you may harm yourself or others, I will call for help."
- "I cannot keep secrets that involve safety risks."

Communication

- "I will not engage in conversations when there is yelling or verbal or physical abuse."

Self-Care

- "I will treat you with respect, and I expect the same."
- "I need time to rest and take care of myself."
- "I cannot be available at all times, but I will help when I can."

Most importantly, caregivers may need to set boundaries for themselves to protect their own well-being. For example, caregivers may need to limit how much time they spend monitoring their loved one in order to create some space and distraction for themselves. Setting boundaries for a loved one might also require setting boundaries for oneself. For example, limiting financial support if a loved one doesn't follow certain treatment recommendations may require fighting an instinct to provide support to one's loved one.

14. Crisis Planning & Higher Levels of Care

Crisis Plan (create when stable)

Creating a plan to address a potential future crisis can help you and your loved one reduce uncertainty, confusion, conflict, and delays in the future. The following guidelines can help you create a crisis plan.

Build the plan

- ☐ Create a crisis plan with your loved one and provider
- ☐ Involve your loved one as much as possible
- ☐ Share the plan with all caregivers and key contacts
- ☐ Review the plan regularly

Key information

- ☐ List current medications, including purpose, doses, side effects
- ☐ Ask prescriber about medication to address acute agitation which can be kept at home and used on an as needed basis
- ☐ List past medications, including purpose, doses, side effects, and reason for discontinuation
- ☐ List past medications that were beneficial
- ☐ List of non-medication treatments such as ECT, TMS and psychotherapy
- ☐ Include history of hospitalizations
- ☐ List key contact and resources for easy reference in a crisis:
    - Emergency contacts
    - Crisis resources (providers, family, friends, 988/911)
    - Current providers
    - Preferred hospitals

Early Actions & Roles

- ☐ Identify early warning signs and triggers
- ☐ Clarify roles (i.e., who does what in a crisis)
- ☐ Designate a trusted family contact your loved one is willing to engage with. Choose someone they trust and communicate with openly

Hospitalization

☐ Review types of hospitalization together (See Part II - Section 3: Types of Hospitalization)

☐ Agree on when to seek hospitalization and type of facility

☐ Agree on specific hospital to visit or admit

Access & Permissions

☐ Keep a copy easily accessible (phone + printed)

☐ Include consent forms or information-sharing permissions if applicable

Learn From Past Crises

☐ Note what helped and didn't

Legal Authorizations

☐ Prepare these documents in advance; consult a lawyer if needed:

- Healthcare Proxy/Medical Power of Attorney: Allows caregiver to make medical decisions in certain situations
- Power of Attorney: Grants broader authority (e.g., financial, legal matters)
- Psychiatric Advance Directive (PAD): Documents your loved one's treatment preferences in advance

Court Interventions (if needed; varies state-by-state)

☐ Guardianship: Court-appointed authority to make personal and medical decisions

☐ Conservatorship: Court-appointed authority to make financial decisions

Peer Respite (an alternative to consider)

Peer respite:

- Offers short term, voluntary, home-like support during a crisis
- Is staffed by people with lived experience rather than clinical staff
- Is not appropriate for situations of acute crisis

☐ Search: "peer respite + your location"

15. How to Communicate

Talking to Your Loved One About Getting Help

☐ Approach with empathy and care
☐ Expect resistance; stigma, denial, and fear are common
☐ Focus on support rather than judgment or blame
☐ Aim to build trust and reduce conflict
☐ Avoid language that feels controlling, dismissive, or shaming
☐ Use calm, clear communication

Active Listening

☐ Rephrase: Restate what you hear in your own words
☐ Clarify: Help them clarify and understand their thoughts
☐ Confirm: Summarize key points to ensure understanding
☐ Explore: Ask open-ended questions and avoid yes/no questions
☐ Share: Offer your perspective calmly and respectfully
☐ Affirm: Validate emotions and acknowledge challenges
☐ Pause intentionally: Give space for your words to land
☐ Allow silence: Create room for reflection
☐ Redirect if needed: Shift or pause if emotions escalate
☐ Assess gently: Explore consequences of inaction without pressure

Discussing Concerns & Involvement in Care

☐ Agree in advance how to raise concerns: Plan how to approach issues when your loved one is not doing well
☐ Agree on responses ahead of time: Draw on what has worked (or not worked) in past episodes
☐ Agree on communication with providers: Clarify when and how you can be involved in care
☐ Revisit agreements when stable: Update based on experience and evolving preferences

Understand Their Concerns

☐ Recognize that your loved one may feel blamed for not doing well

☐ Recognize fear of punishment or loss of control
☐ Recognize fear of treatment changes such as medication changes or hospitalization

Communication Approach
☐ Ask permission Before Involving Others: Respect privacy when discussing their bipolar
☐ Be transparent: Clarify who you may speak with and why
☐ Emphasize support instead of control
☐ Do not expect insight in the moment: Your loved one may not recognize when their thinking is unreasonable
☐ Avoid trying to "talk them out of it"
☐ Shift the conversation to what matters most

Involving Others
☐ Consider involving trusted people, family or friends, with your loved one's permission
☐ Use shared support to reduce isolation and distribute responsibility
☐ Be mindful of your loved one's sensitivity to other people knowing details of their condition, which can be a high-conflict area

Mindset
☐ Respect your loved one's privacy and autonomy
☐ Involve yourself as much as appropriate—but not beyond their comfort
☐ Build trust over time—trust increases openness and willingness to accept help
☐ Reframe negative thinking by helping your loved one consider alternative explanations for problems that feel unsolvable.
☐ Reinforce concepts learned in CBT → See Part II - Section 7
☐ Avoid taking on the role of therapist.

16. Monitoring & Prevention

Caregiver Role

☐ Encourage your loved one to use mood charting and other tracking methods to monitor mood and symptom changes; this record can help empower your loved one

☐ Share observations early and supportively

☐ Review trends together when stable

☐ Develop an understanding of your loved one's triggers

☐ Act as your loved one's early warning system

☐ Act early when warning signs appear

Why It Matters

- Helps detect early warning signs and prevent episodes
- Enables faster response to changes, especially when starting or changing medications
- Provides a record of to show your loved one they've made it through difficult times before

What to Track

☐ Mood (high, low, stable)

☐ Sleep patterns (most important indicator)

☐ Energy and activity levels

☐ Medication adherence and side effects

☐ Stressors and triggers

☐ Menstrual cycle

Tools

☐ Use mood charts to track patterns over time

☐ Consider mood tracking apps (e.g., eMoods or Moodfit)

☐ Consider technologies to track sleep (e.g., Oura rings, Actigraphs or smart phone apps)

☐ Explore structured tools like WRAP (Wellness Recovery Action Plan)

Best Practices

☐ Monitor consistently (daily if possible)

☐ Review patterns together when stable

☐ Use insights to adjust care and prevent escalation

☐ Share data with providers to inform treatment

Daily Monitoring – Key Questions

☐ What does a "good day" look like for your loved one?

☐ Are there any changes from their baseline today?

☐ How is their sleep? *(Sleep is the most important indicator; consider using a tracking device to objectively measure sleep patterns and help disagreements or uncertainties)*

☐ Is there any increase in irritability, energy, or withdrawal?

☐ Are there any medication changes, missed doses, or side effects to note?

Triggers & Patterns

☐ Identify recent triggers (stress, sleep changes, substance use, life events), keeping in mind that:

- Triggers can be positive or negative
- Some episodes occur without clear triggers
- Triggers can repeat

Impact of Self-Stigma on Triggers

☐ Recognize self-stigma can intensify triggers and make them harder to manage

☐ Do not reinforce shame; respond with validation instead

☐ Reduce pressure and judgment

What to Watch For

☐ Disrupted sleep (early warning sign)

☐ Increased stress from relationships, work, or major life changes

☐ Substance use

Prevention & Planning

☐ Track patterns over time, triggers often repeat

☐ Discuss triggers and coping strategies when your loved one is well

☐ Adjust routines or supports to reduce known triggers

Caregiver Awareness

Avoid Mislabeling Symptoms

☐ Do not assume all increased energy or positive mood is hypomania; improvement after depression can look similar

☐ Know your loved one's "normal" (baseline personality) and avoid labeling normal emotions as symptoms, as mislabeling can be discouraging and harm trust

☐ Focus on patterns and functional impact, not isolated moments

☐ Distinguish between the person vs. the illness

Balance Attention Across Episodes

☐ Monitor both mania/hypomania and depression closely

☐ Respond early to changes in either direction

☐ Recognize: mania can lead to serious consequences (e.g., risky behavior)

☐ Recognize: depression carries life-threatening risk (including suicide)

☐ Give equal attention and urgency to both phases

☐ Recognize you may unintentionally trigger symptoms and that stigma can increase sensitivity to everyday comments

☐ Avoid blame or punishment for symptoms beyond their control

Early Warning Signs

☐ Learn your loved one's specific early warning signs. Caregivers may notice changes before the individual does

☐ Watch for reduced need for sleep (most important)

☐ Monitor changes in mood, energy, or behavior

☐ Do they have a shorter fuse than usual

☐ Are they more withdrawn

☐ Less engaged in activities
☐ Do they seem overly animated, dominating a conversation

Coping Strategies

There is no one-size-fits-all approach:

☐ Use a combination of strategies
☐ Know what helps and what makes things worse
☐ Match strategies to the trigger (e.g., stress, sleep, substance use)
☐ Adjust based on severity and duration of symptoms
☐ Expect that sequential treatment efforts may be necessary to find out what works best

Other tips:

☐ Brainstorm coping strategies together with your loved one
☐ While eliminating triggers is ideal, focus on reducing their impact when elimination is not possible
☐ Work with your loved one to help regulate and reduce their emotional response; emotional coping is one of the most effective strategies since emotional response plays a key role in how strongly a trigger affects your loved one.

17. Ready to Pursue Recovery?

Understand the Recovery Framework

☐ Prioritize recovery, not just stability; stability is the starting point, not the goal

☐ Define recovery broadly: a full, meaningful life as your loved one defines it, which may include work and social functioning, financial stability, engagement in family and community, and optimal quality of life

☐ Remember that recovery is not a cure; it is ongoing, requires active management, and follows a non-linear path; setbacks are common and should be expected

☐ Start early: earlier intervention improves long-term outcomes

☐ Know SAMHSA's Working Definition of Recovery https://library.samhsa.gov/product/samhsas-working-definition-recovery/pep12-recdef

Set the Direction

☐ Ask providers to talk about recovery, not just symptom control

☐ Ask providers to treat with recovery as the goal

☐ Talk about the future; focusing on dreams, goals, and what's possible

☐ Show examples of recovery (e.g., advocates, authors, and others living well with bipolar disorder)

☐ Consider additional support (e.g., peer support, bipolar coaching) to build skills and maintain progress

Build the Foundation

☐ Support your loved one but remember you cannot do the work, your loved one needs to take responsibility

☐ Build the right treatment team; keep searching until the fit is right

☐ Create a crisis plan together; preparation builds stability and confidence

Focus on What Matters Most

☐ Prioritize meaning and purpose; support identity, goals, and direction, not just symptoms

☐ Support quality of life by focusing on daily functioning and fulfillment

☐ Encourage independent living skills, including housing, consistent routines, and self-sufficiency

☐ Strengthen relationships by maintaining connection with friends, family, and community

Mindset

☐ Be realistic but not pessimistic; hold onto hope, even when progress is slow

☐ Allow dignity of risk and avoid overprotection, as growth requires trial and error

☐ Reconnect your loved one to their past hopes and dreams, which may still be achievable

☐ Never lose hope

Identity & Strengths: Sources of Pride in Bipolar

☐ Recognize strengths associated with bipolar disorder: Many people experience high levels of creativity, insight, and emotional depth

☐ Use strengths to build self-esteem: Focusing on strengths can counter self-stigma and improve confidence

☐ Highlight positive identity, not just illness: Bipolar disorder is part of the person, not the whole person

☐ Explore examples of creativity and achievement: *Touched with Fire* by Kay Redfield Jamison examines the link between bipolar disorder and creativity

18. Healthy Lifestyle

Sleep

Monitor Sleep
☐ Watch for reduced need for sleep without fatigue, which may indicate hypomania, mania, or medication effect
☐ Watch for excessive sleep, which may indicate depression or a medication effect
☐ Treat any changes in sleep as an early warning sign

Support Healthy Sleep
☐ Encourage consistent sleep schedule with the same bedtime and wake time each day
☐ Practice good sleep hygiene, such as limiting screens, caffeine, and stimulation before bed
☐ Create a calm, low-stimulation sleep environment

Respond to Changes
☐ Contact your loved one's prescriber if sleep changes, as this may signal an emerging episode
☐ Address any medication side effects that affect sleep
☐ Limit alcohol and substances that disrupt sleep

Caregiver Role
☐ Model healthy sleep habits
☐ Reinforce the importance of sleep for stability

See the National Sleep Foundation for more information.

Diet

Awareness
☐ Recognize diet can be affected by medication in several ways:
- Weight changes are a common side effect

- Some medications stimulate appetite and can cause weight gain; if this occurs, have your loved one discuss dietary strategies with their provider
- Altered absorption or tolerability; some medications are better taken with food, so ask your provider

☐ Be aware of dietary considerations that may interact with medication:
- Ask your loved one's provider whether medications have specific food restrictions
- Use caution with diet plans that may influence mood, such as the ketogenic diet, which has not yet been fully studied
- Discuss plans for fasting or intermittent fasting with your loved one's provider in advance

Management
☐ Discuss nutrition and side effects with your loved one's prescriber
☐ Adjust diet to support overall health and stability
☐ Monitor changes in appetite or weight

Support
☐ Consider working with a nutrition expert or dietitian
☐ Create a simple, sustainable meal plan
☐ Encourage regular, balanced meals
☐ Model healthy eating habits

See U.S. Department of Agriculture (MyPlate and Dietary Guidelines) for more information.

Exercise

Benefits
Note: exercise may be hard to initiate when depressed due to a lack of motivation
☐ Proven first-line treatment for mild to moderate depression
☐ Helps offset a sedentary lifestyle

☐ Supports mood, energy, and overall health
Getting Started
☐ Start simple (e.g., short daily walks)
☐ Focus on low-effort, manageable activities
☐ Build consistency over intensity

Support
☐ Consider working with a trainer or structured program for motivation
☐ Exercise together when possible and act as an accountability buddy; involve others if it feels supportive, not pressured
☐ Adjust activity based on energy levels and symptoms
☐ Explore both in-person and online options, such as the Nike Training Club
☐ Use a smartphone app to track outcomes, which can serve as an added incentive

See the CDC (Centers for Disease Control and Prevention) for more information.

Stress Management

Options
☐ Explore different stress management strategies, what works varies by person
☐ Consider meditation, which is widely used and effective

Tools
☐ Use apps to support stress management
☐ Consider evidence-based programs (e.g., UCLA-developed mindfulness tools)

Practice
☐ Build stress management into your loved one's daily routine
☐ Use the listed strategies early, before stress escalates

Good relationships

☐ Model healthy behavior

☐ Surround your loved with people who also maintain healthy relationships

☐ Be an accountability partner, not a controlling presence

☐ Offer support without pressure and focus on overall wellness, not "fixing"

☐ Encourage connections with friends and family; if your loved one is worried about upsetting or triggering you, they may feel safer opening up to others

Complementary & Integrative Health

☐ Discuss any complementary approaches with your treatment provider to ensure they are safe and aligned with your treatment plan

☐ Consider mindfulness, which is especially helpful for stress and symptom management

☐ Use complementary approaches as a support for treatment, not a replacement

Substance Use

☐ Be aware that substances, which are often used to self-medicate or intensify moods, may adversely impact treatment

☐ Limit access to substances in the home and monitor how money or allowances are being spent

☐ Encourage your loved one to attend a support group such as Alcoholics Anonymous or Narcotics Anonymous; consider attending a parallel support group yourself, such as Al-Anon or Nar-Anon.

☐ Consider seeing a therapist with expertise in motivational interviewing

☐ Consider independent treatment for alcohol and substance use disorders

☐ Be aware that certain medications are not safe to combine with certain controlled substances

19. Routine & Environment

Routine & Daily Structure

☐ Maintain a consistent daily routine, covering sleep, meals, and activities

☐ Help your loved one build a daily plan, as lack of structure can worsen depression

☐ Keep regular sleep and wake times, which are the most important elements of routine

☐ Plan simple, predictable daily activities and balance activity and rest; avoiding extremes in either direction

☐ Be aware that sleep deprivation or crossing time zones can dysregulate mood

☐ Ensure your loved one is maintaining basic hygiene and physical self-care

Support Stability

☐ Reduce sudden changes in schedule when possible

☐ Use routines to manage stress and prevent episodes

☐ Build structure around key priorities: Sleep, medication, meals

Caregiver Role

☐ Encourage consistency without being controlling

☐ Help create and reinforce simple routines

☐ Adjust expectations during episodes

Create a Supportive Environment

☐ Maintain a calm, low-stimulation environment during episodes or after hospitalization

☐ Reduce noise, stress, and demands when symptoms are elevated

Practical Support

☐ Help with daily tasks such as cooking, cleaning, and finances when motivation is low

☐ Step in where needed to reduce overwhelm and maintain stability

☐ Offer to do things with your loved one rather than for them when possible

☐ Find opportunities to make your loved one feel needed or useful

Communication Approach

☐ Use supportive, direct language (e.g., "I need your help with this")

☐ Focus on collaboration rather than pressure or criticism

Set Expectations

☐ Keep expectations realistic to avoid overwhelm

☐ Break tasks into small, manageable steps

☐ Create simple, achievable plans for change

☐ Remember that even basic tasks can feel difficult during episodes

Caregiver Role

☐ Model healthy behaviors and routines

☐ Gently and consistently encourage your loved one to maintain social contacts to avoid isolation and foster support

☐ Use gentle encouragement instead of force or pressure

☐ Help your loved one explore the benefits of self-care (e.g., by weighing pros and cons together)

20. Community & Functional Life

Education

☐ Recognize that high-pressure academic environments and social isolation, which often occurs in these environments, are common triggers

☐ Encourage your loved one to choose a college close to home or where they already have a strong support network and seek accommodations

Challenges & Awareness

☐ Expect academic disruptions, including challenges with starting, continuing, or returning to school as mental illness can affect academic progress

Accommodations & Support

☐ Request accommodations through the Office of Disabilities

☐ Use ADA protections (e.g., extended time, flexible deadlines, reduced course load)

☐ Communicate with school support services early

Flexible Options

☐ Reduce course load when needed

☐ Consider online courses, which can be especially helpful during depression

☐ Explore less stressful or local programs to stay close to home

Medical Leave

☐ Have your loved one take an official medical leave if needed (through the school)

☐ Work with your loved one to create a plan for returning before taking leave

☐ Encourage your loved one to avoid dropping out without formal leave when possible

Staying Engaged

☐ Use flexible options to maintain connection to education

☐ Aim to support eventual return to full-time study

Resources

☐ Explore scholarships

☐ Use Clubhouses and community programs for educational support

Employment

Reality & Barriers

☐ Recognize unemployment and underemployment are common in bipolar disorder, often due to symptoms and stigma

☐ Recognize common barriers, including:

- Impact of symptoms on functioning
- Gaps or inconsistencies in work history
- Fear of explaining past experiences to employers
- Feeling the need to start over
- Stigma in the workplace

Focus on Recovery & Support

☐ Prioritize treatment, stability, and stress management

☐ Use the right supports to improve ability to work, as employment outcomes can improve over time

☐ Encourage your loved one to work with qualified professionals for job coaching, resume writing, and interview preparation

Mindset & Motivation

☐ Hold a high bar, as meaningful, productive work is possible

☐ Reinforce strengths (e.g., creativity, resilience, and drive)

☐ Share examples of success, as many professionals live well with bipolar disorder

☐ Encourage hope and confidence

Communication Approach

☐ Be thoughtful when discussing work

☐ Offer support without lowering expectations or limiting ambition
☐ Avoid language that implies incapability

Workplace Accommodations (ADA)

☐ Encourage your loved one to request reasonable accommodations if needed but advise them to carefully consider whether to disclose condition due to stigma. Examples include:

- Flexible schedule
- Quiet workspace
- Time off for appointments

Supported Employment

Supported employment programs help individuals with mental health conditions or disabilities find and maintain competitive jobs by offering structured support in real-world work settings.

☐ Search local programs (e.g., "supported employment + your location")
☐ Check with CCBHCs for referrals

Individual Placement & Support (IPS)

IPS is an evidence-based supported employment model that focuses on rapid job placement in competitive employment. It provides ongoing, individualized long-term support and integrates employment with mental health treatment.

☐ Ask CCBHCs or providers about IPS programs

Additional Options & Supports

☐ Consider lower-stress roles when appropriate (without limiting long-term goals)
☐ Consider part-time and remote work options
☐ Offer to help gather references for your loved one's job search
☐ Encourage volunteer work to build skills and obtain references
☐ Explore Clubhouse programs and community programs for employment support
☐ Don't compare your loved one to others

Supported Housing

Supported housing provides affordable housing with integrated support services while promoting stability, autonomy, and dignity. It is a critical foundation for recovery.

☐ Check with CCBHCs or local programs for availability of supported housing

21. Criminal Justice Involvement

Awareness

☐ Recognize involvement with the criminal justice system can occur during episodes, often involving misdemeanors

☐ Consider whether the incident may reflect a treatment or medication issue

☐ Prioritize diversion to mental health court when possible

Immediate Actions

☐ Stay calm and focused

☐ Contact an attorney, preferably with mental health experience

☐ Inform authorities of your loved one's diagnosis and provide documentation if available

☐ Contact the treatment team as soon as possible

Legal Process

☐ Attend all court proceedings, including competency hearings if applicable

☐ Explore diversion programs or mental health court options

☐ Consider guardianship or conservatorship if appropriate

Legal Support

☐ Seek the best legal advice you can access

☐ Explore legal aid clinics at local law schools

☐ Use state bar association referral services

☐ Consider private attorneys, such as those listed in the Martindale-Hubbell directory for mental health law

☐ Review advocacy resources, such as Bazelon Center for Mental Health Law

22. Estate Planning

Special Needs Trust

☐ Establish a special needs trust to protect eligibility for government benefits, this will:

- Allow assets to be managed without disqualifying the individual from benefits
- Provide long-term financial security

Next Steps

☐ Consult an attorney experienced in disability or estate planning

☐ Ensure the trust is set up correctly to avoid affecting benefits eligibility

23. Homelessness

Awareness

☐ Recognize homelessness risk is higher when treatment is refused or living situations are unstable, and that high-conflict environments can further increase that risk

Prevention

☐ Prioritize stable, supportive housing whenever possible

☐ Address conflicts early to reduce risk of housing loss

☐ Stay engaged, do not withdraw support during difficult periods

Support

☐ Seek help from community resources (e.g., CCBHCs, housing programs)

☐ Explore supportive housing options if needed

24. Ongoing Care & Caregiver Role

Your ongoing care and support are critical for recovery.

Support & Mindset

☐ Lead with hope
☐ Reduce stigma
☐ Make the illness the enemy not your loved one
☐ Tell them you love them, consistently
☐ Help your loved one build self-worth and reinforce identity beyond illness
☐ Remind them that what matters most about them has not changed
☐ Validate emotions, even when they seem unreasonable, as self-stigma may be at play
☐ Encourage acceptance, which is often necessary for recovery
☐ Set high expectations and do not let bipolar disorder lower what your loved one strives for
☐ Recognize that you can provide support but cannot control outcomes
☐ Ask your loved one what they do and don't want you to do; if they're unsure or silent, gently offer support with specific things they may need
☐ Don't assume laziness; self-sabotage (nonadherence, substance use, poor self-care) often reflects low self-worth and need for support
☐ Share stories of others with lived experience to show that recovery is possible
☐ Share facts (e.g., ~7 million people live with bipolar disorder)
☐ Reassure loved one that you love them and will not abandon them

Grief & Acceptance

☐ Allow space to mourn, for both of you, as bipolar disorder can change goals and life paths
☐ Accept shifting timelines and expectations
☐ Focus on what is still possible
☐ Be mindful that your loved one can sense your disappointment

Empowerment & Communication

☐ Empower rather than control; work together and show confidence in your loved one

☐ Involve them in decisions unless they are incapacitated

☐ Ask what helps and what doesn't

☐ Offer practical help (meals, laundry, daily tasks) and be specific about how you will help

☐ Tell them what reduces your worry (e.g., "I'd worry less if you told me when you've taken your medication")

☐ Limit constant talk about bipolar disorder and don't let it define your relationship or their identity

☐ Encourage pursuit of activities unrelated to their illness

☐ Discuss past episodes if they want to

☐ Don't assume they don't care

Daily Support & Engagement

☐ Stay engaged and don't withdraw to avoid conflict

☐ Recognize small wins

☐ Help with tasks during depressive episodes

☐ Don't let your loved one push you away during mania

☐ Recognize that your loved one can't always control symptoms; telling them to stop isn't helpful

☐ Monitor both poles, as depression can be life-threatening

Modeling & Practical Support

☐ Model healthy habits by sleeping, exercising, and eating well together

☐ Stay informed about bipolar disorder and reinforce recovery-oriented principles
→ See Part III: Section 17: Ready to Pursue Recovery

☐ Advocate for excellent care by helping find strong providers and asking providers treatment when appropriate

Social Support & Advocacy

☐ Connect your loved one to peer support, communities, nonprofits with lived experience

☐ Educate others about bipolar disorder, but never share their condition without their consent

☐ Expand their support network, help them feel less like a burden and preserve relationships to reduce isolation

☐ With permission, explain their situation to others

Safety & Reality of Illness

☐ Recognize that suffering can exist even when your loved one seems well, as self-stigma is painful even when not visible

☐ Prioritize safety, mania can involve anger or violence, especially when substances are involved

Talking About the Past (Use Carefully)

☐ Avoid harmful comparisons and don't emphasize who they used to be

☐ Use the past constructively to remind them of their true identity and strengths

Most Important

☐ Never assume your loved one doesn't care

25. Caregiver Self-care: You Matter Too

☐ Be aware of stigma and your own biases
☐ Educate yourself about bipolar disorder
☐ Advocate for both your loved one and yourself
☐ Build communication and de-escalation skills
☐ Prioritize your own self-care, including your own mental health, and take regular breaks and use support groups
☐ Set and maintain boundaries, and know when to say no
☐ Do not ignore your own needs; seek professional support if needed
☐ Maintain your support system by staying connected to friends, family, and community
☐ Use available benefits and resources such as FMLA (Family and Medical Leave Act), EAP (Employee Assistance Program), and other workplace supports)
☐ Recognize strengths often seen in people with bipolar disorder; many are empathetic, creative, and resilient
☐ Avoid self-blame, as it can lead to second-guessing your decisions and your ability to help your loved one

26. Top 10 Mistakes Caregivers Make

- **Assuming your loved one doesn't care:** This is often a symptom of depression or lack of insight, not a lack of love or effort
- **Stopping at stability instead of aiming for recovery:** Stability is the floor, not the goal
- **Setting expectations too low:** This can limit independence and reinforce illness identity
- **Taking control instead of building collaboration:** This may create resistance and damage trust
- **Focusing only on the illness, not the person:** This can erode identity and self-worth
- **Dwelling on past episodes:** This often increases shame and reduces openness
- **Not advocating enough:** Poor care often continues unless challenged
- **Relying only on professionals:** Your role matters more than you think, and a team approach that includes those with lived experience is invaluable
- **Not asking what they want:** This reduces buy-in and increases resistance
- **Blaming yourself:** Bipolar disorder is not caused by caregivers

Most caregivers make some of these mistakes, but awareness helps you respond more effectively

Finally, love will always be stronger than bipolar disorder

27. When You Need More Support

Also from Katherine Ponte

Ponte, K and Goncalves, I. (2025). *Loving Someone with a Serious Mental Illness: Caring for Your Loved One and Yourself on the Journey to Mental Health Recovery.* New Harbinger Publications.

Ponte. K. (2023). *Your Mental Health Recovery Workbook: Sharing Hope for Recovery,* Original publisher: Trigger Publishing. Updated edition. Self-published.

Ponte. K. (2022). *ForLikeMinds: Mental Illness Recovery Insights*. Self-published. Named a book of note for recovery by the National Alliance on Mental Illness' *You Are Not Alone*.

HELPFUL BOOKS

***The Bipolar Checklist* is not a replacement for these excellent books. It's a practical companion.**

Amador, X (2022). *I Am Not Sick I Don't Need Help!: How to Help Someone Accept Treatment*. Vida Press.

Daramus, A. (2020). *Understanding Bipolar Disorder: The Essential Family Guide.* Callisto Publishing.

Duckworth, K. (2022). *You Are Not Alone: The NAMI Guide to Navigating Mental Health-With Advice from Experts and Wisdom from Real People and Families*. Zando Publishing.

Fast, J. and Preston, J. (2023). *Take Charge of Bipolar Disorder: A 4-Step Plan for You and Your Loved Ones to Manage the Illness and Create Lasting Stability*. Balance Publishing.

Fast, J. and Preston, J. (2012). *Loving Someone with Bipolar Disorder: Understanding and Helping Your Partner*. New Harbinger Publications.

Miklowitz, D. (2024). *Living Well with Bipolar Disorder: Practical Strategies for Improving Your Daily Life.* The Guilford Press.

Miklowitz, D. (2019). *The Bipolar Disorder Survival Guide: What You and Your Family Need to Know.* The Guilford Press.

Mondimore, F. (2020). *Bipolar Disorder: A Guide for You and Your Loved Ones.* Johns Hopkins University Press.

Ponte, K and Goncalves, I. (2025). *Loving Someone with a Serious Mental Illness: Caring for Your Loved One and Yourself on the Journey to Mental Health Recovery.* New Harbinger Publications.

NONPROFIT ORGANIZATIONS

General mental health nonprofits offer accessible resources, education, and community support that can benefit people with bipolar disorder. They provide guidance on coping, self-care, and treatment, and help reduce isolation through peer support and advocacy. Ask your friends and family and providers for recommendations.

National Alliance on Mental Illness (NAMI) and over 650 state and local affiliate organizations
Active Minds
American Foundation for Suicide Prevention
Clubhouse International
Depression and Bipolar Support Alliance and +150 chapters
Fountain House
Heinz C. Prechter Bipolar Research Program
International Bipolar Foundation
International Society for Bipolar Disorders
Mental Health America and its nationwide network of 240 affiliates
National Federation of Families and approximately 115 affiliate organizations
Ryan Licht Sang Bipolar Foundation
Substance Use and Mental Health Services Administration (SAMHSA)
Trevor Project

PROVIDER DIRECTORIES

The best referrals often come from friends, family, and healthcare providers.

Finding the right providers can be one of the biggest challenges and it may take trying a few before finding the best fit.

These directories can feel overwhelming, but they expand options and can help connect you with culturally competent providers. Better fit leads to stronger engagement, trust, and outcomes.

We do not endorse specific directories. Review each one carefully and exercise caution.

Top Starting Points

☐ American Psychiatric Association (psychiatrists)
☐ American Psychological Association (psychologists)
☐ American Society of Clinical Psychopharmacology (psychiatrists)
☐ Psychology Today (therapists)
☐ SAMHSA Early Serious Mental Illness Treatment Locator (psychosis)
☐ SAMHSA Treatment Locator findtreatment.gov (treatment centers)

Other psychiatry focused

☐ American Academy of Addiction Psychiatry
☐ Association of Gay and Lesbian Psychiatrists

Other therapy focused

☐ American Association for Marriage and Family Therapy
☐ American Counseling Association
☐ National Association of Social Workers

Culturally Competent Care

☐ Asian Mental Health Collective

☐ Association of Black Psychologist
☐ Inclusive Therapists
☐ Latinx Therapy
☐ LGBTQ+ Psychotherapists of Color Directory
☐ National Queer and Trans Therapists of Color Network
☐ Therapy for Black Girls
☐ Therapy for Black Men

$ Low-Cost/Accessible Options
☐ SAMHSA Treatment Locator
☐ Open Path Psychotherapy Collective
☐ Community mental health centers (via NAMI affiliates)

Katherine Ponte

Katherine is an award-winning mental health advocate, best-selling author and Assistant Clinical Professor of Psychiatry at the Yale School of Medicine. She is the author of *Loving Someone with a Serious Mental Illness*, published by New Harbinger, *Your Mental Health Recovery Workbook: Sharing Hope for Recovery* and *ForLikeMinds: Mental Illness Recovery Insights*. She is the founder of Bipolar Thriving: Bipolar Recovery Coaching and Psych Ward Greeting Cards, a leading psychiatric hospital outreach nonprofit. Katherine is also a Certified Psychiatric Rehabilitation Practitioner, and a New York Certified Peer Specialist-Provisional. She built the ForLikeMinds mental health peer support platform into a community of over 150,000 members that has reached millions with resources and insights. She is a lawyer and has a graduate degree from the University of Pennsylvania and is a board member of the National Alliance on Mental Illness–NYC.

Katherine has been living with severe bipolar I disorder with psychosis, including extended periods of suicidal depression, for over 25 years and reached recovery in 2018. She is the recipient of the highest honor in the bipolar disorder community, the Mogens Schou Award from the International Society for Bipolar Disorders, and one of the highest mental health honors in New York City, NAMI-NYC's Ending the Silence Award.

Katherine is based in New York City and the Catskills, where she lives with her spouse and tremendous supporter, Izzy, and their adorable British shorthair, Mel, and irresistible frenchie, Lu.

Joseph F. Goldberg

Dr. Goldberg, M.D. is a Clinical Professor of Psychiatry at the Icahn School of Medicine at Mount Sinai in New York, Immediate-Past President, American Society of Clinical Psychopharmacology and Deputy Editor-in-Chief, The Journal of Clinical Psychiatry. He has been in private practice with a focus on mood disorders for 30 years and is the author of over 250 publications, including the best-selling book *Managing the Side Effects of Psychotropic Medications* published by American Psychiatric Publications.

www.ingramcontent.com/pod-product-compliance
Lightning Source LLC
LaVergne TN
LVHW010737061126
851857LV00014B/1513
* 9 7 9 8 2 3 4 1 5 7 7 6 8 *